Top Nutritional Supplement Buying Guide

Series 2: Muscle Building

Written by
Daniel Lee Staneart

Contents

Intro to the Supplement Guide

This supplement buying guide is Series 2, which will reveal and list top muscle building supplements. If you've read Series 1, then you read about my top supplements for general overall health and wellness.

The area of muscle building with weights and supplements is where I first started gaining knowledge about dietary supplements beginning in 1993. I was 19 years old, extremely skinny weighing only around 125 lbs at a height of 6 feet. So, you could imagine my slender appearance.

I was tired of being told how skinny I was all the time as well as having an embarrassing nickname. I didn't have much self-confidence as you might have guessed, and was already kind of shy to begin with, especially when it came to approaching or talking to girls.

So, here's my short testimony ...

I wanted to change my body as well as make it stronger. I received my first weight bench set with concrete plates when I was 12, but they never really would get used until seven years later. I started lifting weights and learning the basics. I gained over 50 lbs of lean mass during the first 8 months of lifting weights, which I started in June of 93'.

After 8 months or so went by people really didn't recognize me, and some even thought that I must have used steroids to change my body the way that I did. By January 1994, I weighed 175 lbs and was pretty much all muscle. I was already very lean so I had a flat stomach to begin with and low body fat percentage. I had such a high metabolism and was eating so much food as well as drinking weight gain shakes to keep my body weight up and muscles growing.

I worked a full-time job making only $3.85 an hour so purchasing steroids wasn't even an option for me. Besides, I wouldn't have had any idea where to even get them. However, I did know of the dangers of anabolic steroids and would have never touched them based on health risks alone.

In a nutshell, this is how I basically put on 50 lbs of lean muscle mass in 8 months:

I only worked out my upper body for the first few months, but I was growing and learning. Keep in mind that I was 19 years old and so my testosterone and growth hormone levels were soaring. I was reading whatever I could find on weightlifting, muscle gaining and nutritional supplements. I first started purchasing muscle building supplements at a GNC store during that time. They always gave me tips and a free muscle magazine each month.

What was my weight lifting routine?

It was kind of sporadic at first concentrating primarily on my arms, but also performing some chest, back and shoulder work. However, I was quickly learning a lot from the free muscle magazines that I was getting, which were Muscle & Fitness, Ironman and I think Muscular Development.

Later on, the best "muscle" magazine that I ever read and starting actually buying and learning so much more from was Muscle Media 2000 represented by EAS (Bill & Shawn Phillips). In late summer 1993, I started purchasing and using weight gain powders, which was the first supplement that I ever bought for myself. I also finally started working out my legs and it made such a big difference. My entire body and muscles grew even more once I started performing squats.

Here is the solid routine I established for myself by the Fall of 93':

<u>3 days on and 1 day off</u>

Day 1:

Chest - 4 sets of flat bench barbell press, 4 sets of incline bench barbell press, 2 sets of dumbbell flyes

Triceps - 6 sets of standing close-grip barbell press, 4 sets of lying close-grip barbell press

Day 2:

Back - 6 to 8 sets of bent-over barbell rows

Biceps - 6 to 8 sets of standing barbell curls

Shoulders - 6 sets of behind-the-nech barbell press, 4 sets of front military barbell press, 4 sets of dumbbell side laterals

Traps - 4 sets of standing barbell shoulder shrugs

Day 3:

Legs - 6 to 8 sets of squats

Day 4:

Off

I would perform anywhere from 8 to 15 reps on every set (exercise) and body part pushing myself past the pain zone. When I worked my traps I actually would perform about 30 reps on each set. On most exercises I always used a weight poundage that made it very hard for me to get 10 reps, then I'd push past that with a couple more forced reps. I normally rested 1 to 2 minutes between each set. When I performed squats I rested about 3 to 5 minutes between sets.

I worked out alone with no spotter, but still lifted with a lot of heart and intensity. I had the kind of mindset that every time I even touched a weight I knew that I would grow putting on new muscle. I stayed completely focused and disciplined. I can even remember puking a few times after doing squats from pushing myself so hard.

Occasionally, I changed my routine up as well to get past those grueling and even boring plateaus. For example, sometimes I would incorporate dumbbell presses into my chest and shoulder routines. Playing music while working out always helped me a lot to.

Back to my routine...

After Day 4, then I would just start my workout regimen all back over again. I made so much progress and gains on this routine, but I was most likely over-training. I was working a full-time job 8-12 hours a day sometimes six days a week, which was a physical hard labor position in the hot Louisiana heat. When I got home from work I would eat and then drink a weight gain shake. I always waited an hour or so after eating before I worked out.

Once I was through lifting, then I would drink another weight gain shake right away or wait about 15 minutes after drinking some juice or water. You have to get some carbs and protein into your body after you workout for maximizing muscle gains as well as recovery. About an hour later after that, I would eat another meal of some sort. We didn't have much so I ate pretty much anything.

I think one of the reasons why I made such good progress is because I was consistent and never missed a workout. I also worked out with a lot of intensity, determination and visualization. I really believed in myself and had faith that I could transform my body. I even remember receiving a couple really tough injuries and bouncing back very quickly both times during the 90's.

One time somebody who knew me in high school asked me how long I had been working out. I said about eight months, during that time, and he couldn't believe it. He wanted to know how I made such big gains because he had been working out for three years. As we starting talking, I asked him how often he changed the amount of weight (pounds) he was lifting.

He said that he'd been lifting the same amount of poundage for about 3 years. I let him know that was the problem. The body adapts to the stress that you put on it, which goes the same for muscle fibers. They get worked, split and grow. If you put the same stress on it every time with no change then they wont grow any further. Basically, you'll stay the same with virtually no new muscle growth.

I don't remember exactly, but I'm pretty sure that I was increasing my weight poundage on every exercise a little bit each month. I was kind of limited though with concrete plates, but I eventually got some steel plates and a better bench. I made my own squat rack out of my first older small bench and rack.

Here are the primary nutritional supplements that I used in the 90's:

Cybergenics Infinity 1700 (Weight Gain Powder), Amino Acid tablets, Vanadyl Sulfate (10 mg), Boron and even Colostrum. I bought all these supplements at GNC during the 90's.

I also tried some other weight gain powders, especially after Cybergenics stopped selling theirs in GNC. I used Mega Mass 2000, Hard-body Gainer 3600 and Muscle-Blast 2000. Needless to say, muscle building supplements have come a long way since the 90's. I wouldn't recommend these supplements today, but amino acid tabs, vanadyl sulfate, boron and colostrum still can be useful in the right high quality form. I'll also add that the taste of 90's weight-gain powders were sometimes very hard to choke down.

Later I believe in 94', the company AST and Prolab starting putting out some decent weight-gain, protein and post-workout powders which I did use as well. The company EAS, owned and operated by Bill Phillips along with Shawn Phillips, came along during this time to and completely changed the muscle building supplement industry with their products, especially creatine. EAS and PROLAB are still successful today putting out great quality supplements.

There were times that I stopped working out for personal reasons but never for longer than 6 months. Even during those times I still worked out when I could, but I just wasn't able to stay consistent. I rebuilt my body again during two other major times in my life that involved change both in 1997 and in 2003. I rebuilt my body one last time in mid to late 2014 at the age of 40, but did stop working out after that this time for over a year because of some injuries and the line of employment that I was working in.

I will say that without a doubt nutritional supplements

really helped me. There's no way that I would have got the calories and protein that I needed to put on the muscle mass I acheived back in 1993-94 without them, especially being what is known as a hard-gainer.

I've always kept up with the nutritional supplement industry even still today. Are you ready to view some top muscle building supplements and where to buy them?

Part 1

Places that sell supplements

This section will be similar to my Series 1 book providing those with valuable information who haven't read the first book yet. There are many stores that sell nutritional supplements.

Some of the most known retail places to shop are GNC, Vitamin World, The Vitamin Shoppe, Super Supplements, CVS, Walgreens, Rite Aid, Target and even Wal-mart. Discovering which supplements are the best, purest, safest and priced fairly definitely takes some research.

There are many online supplement stores available on the internet. Some of the top and my personal favorites that I shop from happen to be wholesale companies. All wholesale nutritional supplement companies sell virtually all known quality brand name supplements as well as their own line of products at a much lower cost than retail.

I try to save more money by shopping for high quality supplement brand names at a much lower wholesale cost. Many times some of the stores listed above, such as GNC, will have some really good sales and bargains as well.

Here are my top three wholesale supplement companies to choose from also mentioned in my Series 1 book as well:

Nutrition Express

Nutrition Express will send you a free catalog by mail or you can go straight to their website. They have a huge selection of quality brand name products as well as their own represented product lines at wholesale prices. Nutrition Express focuses on overall health, weight-loss and muscle building. They also always offer tips, advice and have excellent articles. Here is their toll free number and website link: 1-800-338-7979 or go to

www.nutritionexpress.com

ProSource

ProSource supplements will send you a free catalog by mail or you can go straight to their website. They have a good selection of quality brand name products as well as their own high quality product line at wholesale prices. ProSource focuses more on muscle building and weight-loss. They also always offer tips, advice, excellent articles and helpful supplement ratings. Here is their toll free number and website link: 1-800-310-1555 or go to www.prosource.net

Swanson Vitamins

Swanson Vitamins will send you a free catalog by mail or you can go straight to their website. They primarily focus on their own Swanson name products, but also have a great selection of quality brand name products at wholesale prices. Swanson Vitamins is a great company for finding unique and herbal supplements and they tend to focus on overall health. They also have good supplement articles, informative videos and customer reviews. Here is their toll free number and website link: 1-800-437-4148 or go to www.swansonvitamins.com

This supplement buying guide is part of a 3-book series. You can purchase Series 1 on Amazon in the ebook or paperback version. This is series 2, which will focus on the top muscle building supplements.

Series 3 will focus on weight loss revealing the top dietary supplements in that category. All three books are top nutritional supplement buying guides.

Hopefully this guide will give you direction in finding the right supplement, brand and price for your needs. I wrote this book to help people and to answer these three questions .... What, Where and How much?

Remember to always consult your doctor before using certain supplements especially if you're taking medications.

Let's get started....

Part 2

Top supplements and brands
to choose

What are some of the top nutritional supplements and brands to choose this new 2016 year to benefit your muscles based on safety, effectiveness, quality and price?

Protein Powders

Protein is a primary ingredient that you cannot go without when it comes to building muscle. You have to get your protein intake from food and or supplemental sources. Protein powder supplements really help you cut down on calories and food intake while ingesting the amount of protein you need to stay lean while building muscle. Protein powders are safe and recommended for both guys and gals.

When looking for protein powders to buy try to find those that contain whey protein, especially concentrate, isolate and peptides. There are literally tons of brands to choose from, but I'm gonna list my top recommended brands:

Next Proteins (Designer Whey), EAS, BSN, Cytosport, ProSource, Fitness Labs, Lindberg, MuscleTech, Optimum Nutrition (ON), Jay Robb, MHP, Gaspari, Labrada, Universal Nutrition, Met-Rx, Nature's Best, NOW Foods, Arnold Schwarzenegger Series, BPI Sports, Ronnie Coleman Signature Series, PROLAB, AST Sports Science and Beverly International.

My top picks for protein powder based on quality, safety and price:

Next Proteins (Designer Whey) brand. You can buy this in 2 or 4 lbs size. The 2 lb offers 32 servings with 18 g of protein per serving. This product is 100% natural and various flavors are offered which taste good. The product image below is gourmet chocolate flavor. Purchase online through Nutrition Express, Prosource or Swanson Vitamins. Prosource offers the best price at $25.95. I'd recommend this product for all ages that desire to use a protein powder. A smaller 12 oz. container of Designer Whey protein is available through Swanson Vitamins.

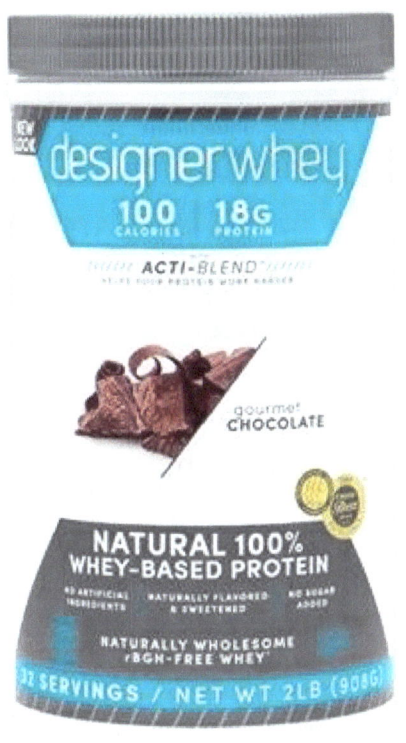

If you prefer a completely unflavored organic whey protein powder then I'd recommend NOW Foods brand. It's a 1 lb container offering 19 servings with 19 g of protein per serving for $24.95. Purchase online through Prosource.

More safe and natural protein powder recommendations:

Fitness Labs and Lindberg Whey Protein or Whey Isolate

are both excellent and really some of the best tasting in my opinion. I'd recommend these protein powders and all other natural protein products listed for all ages who desire to use a dietary protein supplement.

Lindberg Whey Protein 2 lb container offering 26 servings with 25 g protein per serving. Various flavors are offered. Lindberg protein is all-natural and taste good. The image below is natural vanilla. Purchase online through Nutrition Express for $24.99. Lindberg also offers this product in a 5 lb and 5 oz. Container.

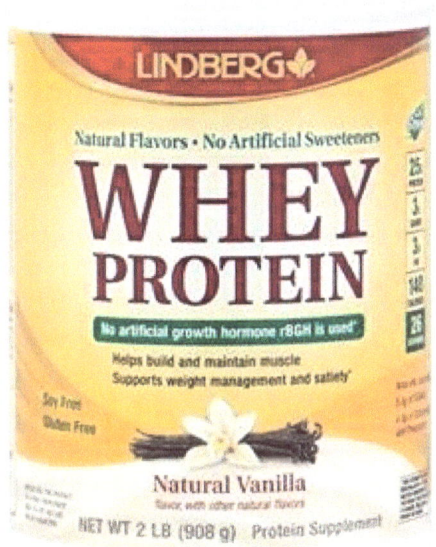

Fitness Labs Wheyfit Isolate 2 lb container offering 29 servings with 25 g protein per serving. Various flavors are offered and the image below is strawberry swirl. Purchase online through Nutrition Express for $30.99. Fitness Labs also offers 5 oz. containers for $5.99

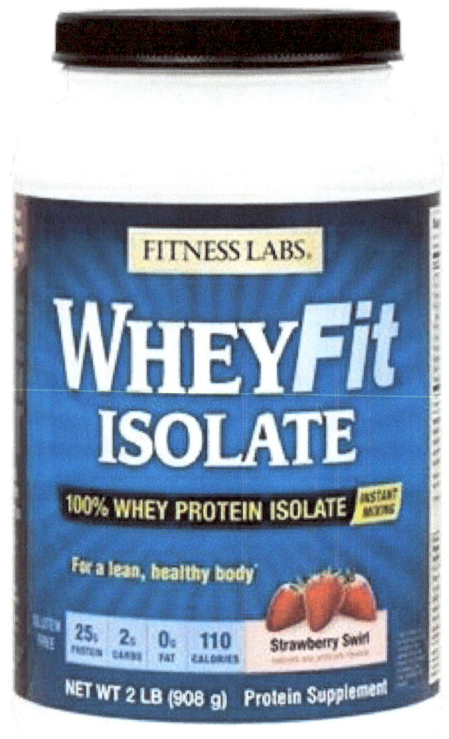

Fitness Labs Musclefit Protein (6-protein blend) 2 lb container offering 27 servings with 25 g protein per serving. Various flavors are offered. Purchase online through Nutrition Express for $24.99

Fitness Labs Wheyfit Protein 2 lb container offering 25 servings with 25 g protein per serving. Various flavors are offered. Purchase online through Nutrition Express for $22.99

All three of these Fitness Labs brand protein come in a 5 lb size as well.

Jay Robb Whey Protein 24 oz bag offering 23 servings with 25 g protein per serving. All-natural and great tasting. Various flavors are offered and the image below is chocolate. Purchase online through Nutrition Express for $37.20

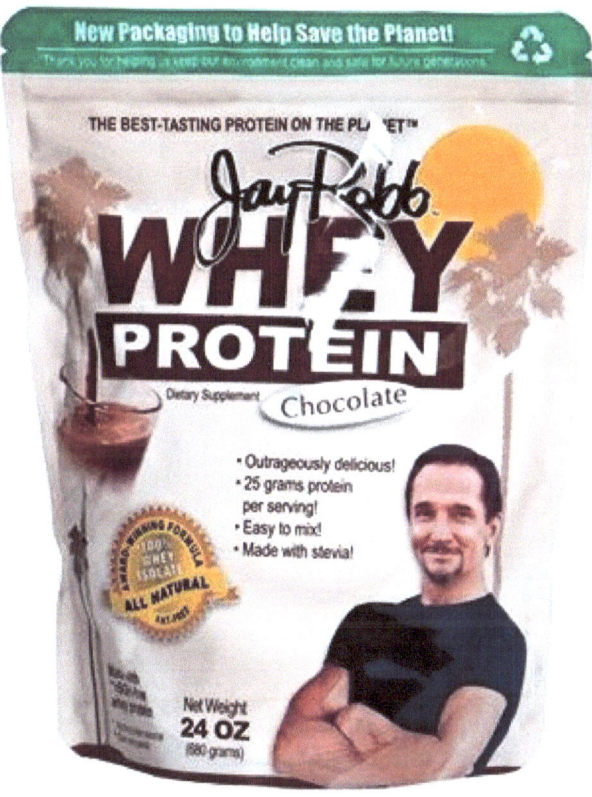

Met-Rx Natural Whey 5 lb container offering 68 servings

with 23 g protein per serving. Various flavors are offered. Purchase online through Prosource for $48.95

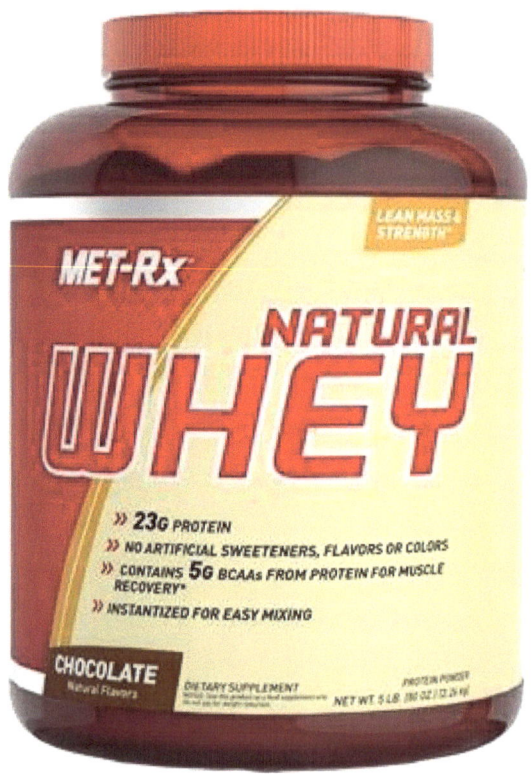

Other high quality whey protein brand recommendations that are not all-natural but produce excellent results:

EAS 100% Whey Protein 5 lb container offering 58 servings with 26 g protein per serving. Various flavors are offered. Purchase online through Nutrition Express for $44.95

Prosource NytroWhey Ultra Elite 2.71 lb container offering 28 servings with 21 g protein per serving. Various flavors are offered. Purchase online through Prosource for $30.50

Optimum Nutrition (ON) Gold Standard 100% Whey 2 lb container offering 29 servings with 24 g protein per serving. Various flavors are offered. Purchase online through Nutrition Express for $29.89

Cytosport Monster Isolate 2.2 lb container offering 30 servings with 25 g protein per serving. Various flavors are offered. Purchase online through Nutrition Express for $29.99

MuscleTech Platinum 100% Whey Protein 2 lb container offering 27 servings with 24 g protein per serving. Various flavors are offered. Purchase online through Nutrition Express for $26.99

MHP Maximum Whey 5 lb container offering 58 servings with 25 g protein per serving. Various flavors are offered. Purchase online through Prosource for $49.95

BSN Syntha 6 Isolate 2 lb container offering 24 servings with 25 g protein per serving. Various flavors are offered. Purchase online through Prosource for $32.25

AST Sports Science VP2 Whey Isolate with Aminogen 2 lb container offering 32 servings with 24 g of protein per serving. Various flavors are offered. Purchase online through Prosource for $37.95

Gaspari Myofusion Advanced Protein 2 lb container offering 24 servings with 25 g protein per serving. Various flavors are offered. Purchase online through Prosource for $30.99

Muscle Building & Recovery

There are many supplements, along with protein powders, that help you build muscle, recover faster, gain strength and help decrease your body-fat percentage. Let's list some of the best...

CREATINE:

Creatine is a chemical naturally produced by our body and is involved in the production of energy which benefits our muscles. Although there are several health benefits from using creatine you must still use it correctly and in moderation. Both guys and gals have used this supplement for its health and muscle benefits throughout the years.

Pure german creatine is known for being the best, but there are so many brands and combinations today. It comes in both powder and capsule form. Creatine improves strength, endurance, recovery, concentration and muscle building. Many of the best brands I've listed for protein powder also are some of the best brands for creatine as well.

My top picks for creatine powder based on quality, safety and price:

Fitness Labs German Creatine (1,000 grams) 2.2 lb container offering 200 servings at 5 g per serving. Pure Creatine (Creapure) with nothing else added. Purchase online through Nutrition Express for $19.99

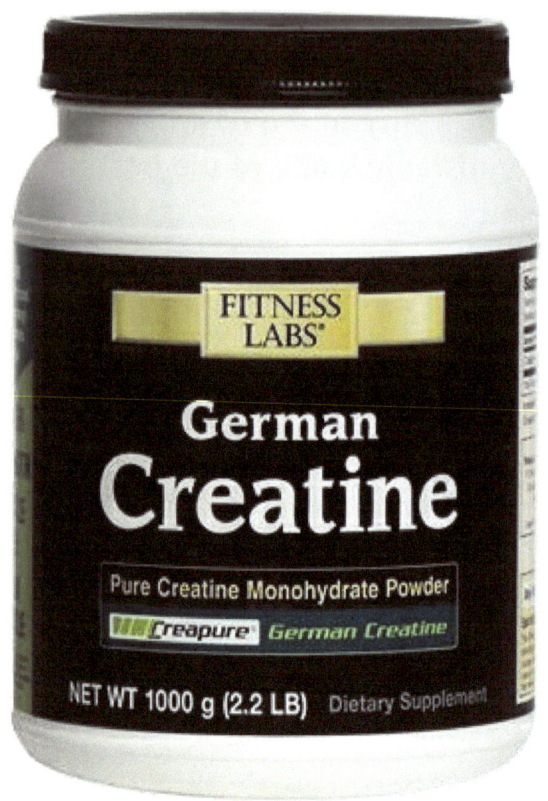

Prosource Creatine Monohydrate 1,000 gram container offering 200 servings at 5 g per serving. Pure Creatine (Creapure) with nothing else added. Purchase online through Prosource for $17.50

Some people prefer micronized creatine, which bascially means that the creatine particles are smaller, finer and do not really settle at the bottom of your cup or shaker when drinking. Fitness Labs offers micronized creatine as well.

Fitness Labs Micronized Creatine (1,000 g) 2.2 lb container offering 200 servings at 5 g per serving. Purchase online through Nutrition Express for $16.99

There are also various beneficial ways to utilize creatine by mixing or combining it with other ingredients. Creatine seems to perform and uptake better in the body when you mix it with juice, such as grape juice. Creatine, along with carbohydrates, is well known for shuttling amino acids (protein) and glucose (carbs) straight into muscle cells, which of course is what you want.

There are so many brands and forms of creatine on the market today that have also combined creatine with other ingredients to make it more potent. Some examples of this would be by combining it with glutamine, taurine, alpha Lipoic acid, phosphates, nitric oxide producers, cinnulin and high-glycemic carbs (dextrose). I normally would just add a teaspoon of pure creatine to my protein shake which also works great.

I try to stay away from supplement products that contain to many unnecessary and even harmful chemicals, additives and food colorings. Here's a good supplemental example pick of creatine combined with other ingredients to increase its potency based on quality, price and safety:

Fitness Labs CreaFit Creatine Transport 4 lb container offering 42 servings at 5 g of creatine per serving along with other combined ingredients. Purchase online through Nutrition Express for $22.99

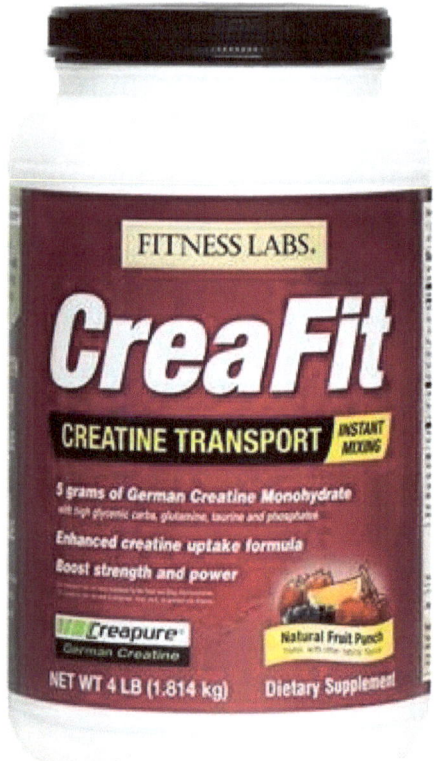

A loading phase for creatine is also normally recommended as well as cycling on and off periods.

L-GLUTAMINE:

Glutamine is one of the most abundant amino acids produced in the body. Glutamine has been used as a treatment for various conditions. It is very beneficial for the immune system, healing and recovery.

Glutamine is an important key and very helpful in the muscle-building process, specifically in the area of recovery. This powerful amino acid is necessary for an anabolic state of muscle growth. It also benefits your growth hormone and energy levels. Many of the best brands I've listed for protein powder also are some of the best brands for glutamine as well. It comes in both powder and convenient capsule form. I wanna also note that most high quality protein powders contain added glutamine and glutamine peptides.

My top picks for glutamine powder based on quality, safety and price:

Fitness Labs L-Glutamine 1 lb container offering 89 servings at 5 g per serving. Pure USP Grade Glutamine. Purchase online through Nutrition Express for $15.99

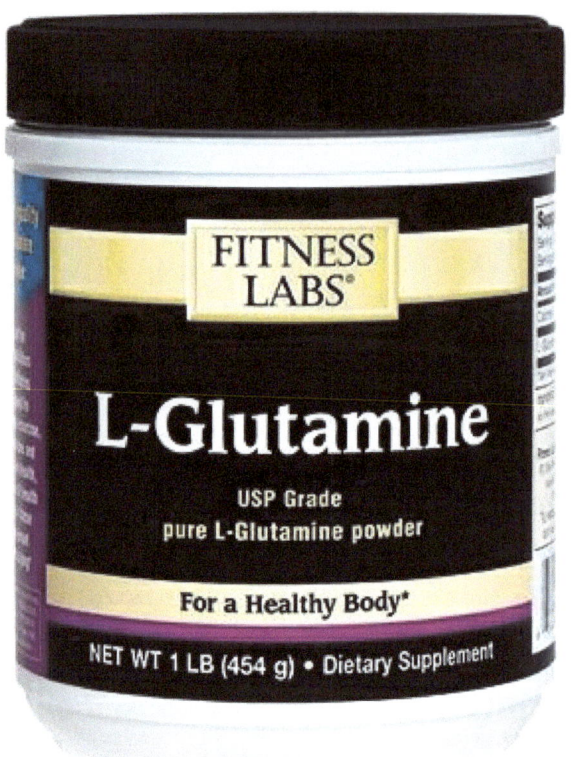

Gaspari Glutamine 300 grams offering 60 servings at 5 g per serving. Pure micronized L-Glutamine. Purchase online through Nutrition Express for $15.89

HMB:

HMB is a metabolite of the branched-chain amino acid leucine. What does it do? Helps prevent protein and muscle breakdown. HMB also supports more efficient muscle growth and recovery. Research studies have revealed that HMB is effective with no side effects.

My top picks for HMB based on quality, safety and price:

Fitness Labs HMB offering 360 caps at 250 mg per capsule. Most research studies show that taking 3 grams of HMB a day is most effective. Purchase online through Nutrition Express for $21.99

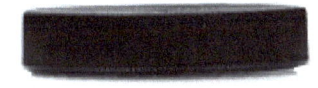

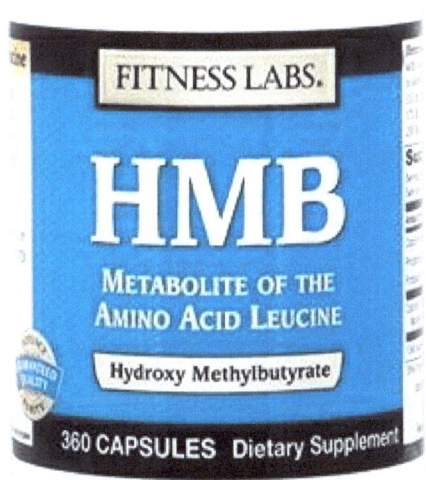

Met-Rx HMB offering 90 caps at 1 g per serving. Purchase online through Prosource for $26.95

Optimum Nutrition HMB offering 90 caps at 1 g per serving. Purchase online through Swanson Vitamins for $30.08

Swanson HMB offering 90 vcaps at 1 g per serving. Purchase online through Swanson Vitamins for $28.99

TESTOSTERONE BOOSTERS:

There are many test boosters on the market today that prove to be very effective. Some of the brands listed for protein powders are some of the best for test boosters as well. What do they do? They raise testosterone levels which benefits sex drive, lean muscle growth, increases strength, faster recovery and a decrease in bodyfat.

What are some of the best ingredients to look for when searching for test booster?

Real test boosters may contain one or some of these ingredients in no particular order: D-Aspartic Acid, Cordyceps Extract, Fenugreek Seed Extract, Sarsaparilla Extract, Eurycoma Longifolia Extract, Nettle Root (Stinging Nettle) Extract, Beta Sitosterol, DIM (Diindolylmethane), Tribulus Terrestris extract, L-Carnitine L-Tartrate (LCLT), Maca Root Extract, Horny Goat Weed (Epimedium Grandiflorum), Turmeric (curcumin), Avena Sativa Extract, Muira Puama, Mucuna Pruriens (L-Dopa), Flax Seed, Polypodium vulgare (20-hydroxyecdysone), Yohimbe Extract, Gensing Extract, Ashwagandha Extract, Boron and Chrysin.

Okay, let's narrow it down ... which of these ingredients are most effective? I would say Fenugreek Seed Extract (Fenusides & Saponins), Eurycoma Longifolia (Glycosaponins & Eurypeptides), Tribulus Terrestris Extract (Saponins & Protodioscin), Curcumin extract and D-Aspartic Acid (DAA). The other above ingredients are beneficial as well and many times combined with the top three or four extracts listed here. Many times D-Aspartic Acid is a standalone supplement. However, you can get any of these ingredients by themselves in supplemental form.

Some of the other ingredients listed above are good tonics and support general health like Sarsaparilla. Also, some of the lesser ingredients listed above, such as DIM and Chrysin, are very beneficial in decreasing and preventing estrogen production in men. It's also not a bad idea to use supplements like Saw Palmetto Extract or Beta-Sitosterol. These actually help reduce harmful DHT, hair-loss and protect the prostate, so these products would definitely benefit men. I also prefer to choose a test booster that doesn't contain no or very little unnecessary added chemicals which can be harmful.

ZMA is another strength and testosterone boosting product that is offered through many brands. It has been tested and proven to be effective. ZMA basically contains Vitamin B-6, Magnesium and Zinc in specific amounts. This supplement works best when taken at bedtime.

My top picks for testosterone boosters based on quality, safety and price:

Fitness Labs Tribulus Ultra offering 90 caps containing 30 servings. This product contains tribulus terrestris extract along with other effective ingredients such as fenugreek extract, eurycoma longifolia extract and more. Purchase online through Nutrition Express for $24.99

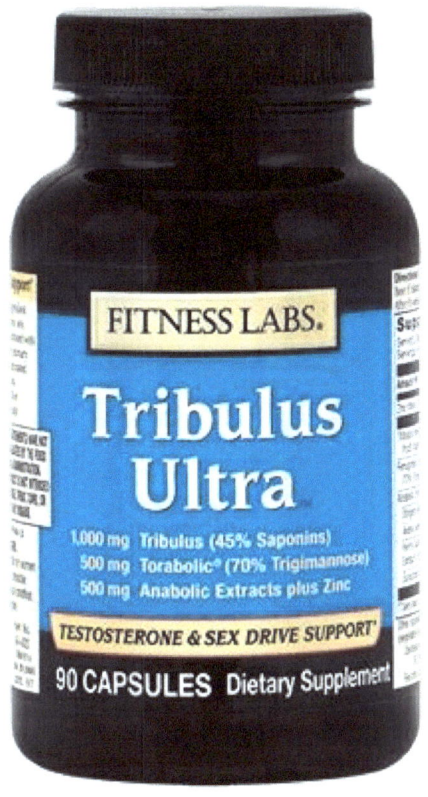

Nature's Plus T Male offering 60 caps containing 30 servings. This supplement contains a great combination of test boosting ingredients and is all natural. Purchase online through Nutrition Express for $22.99

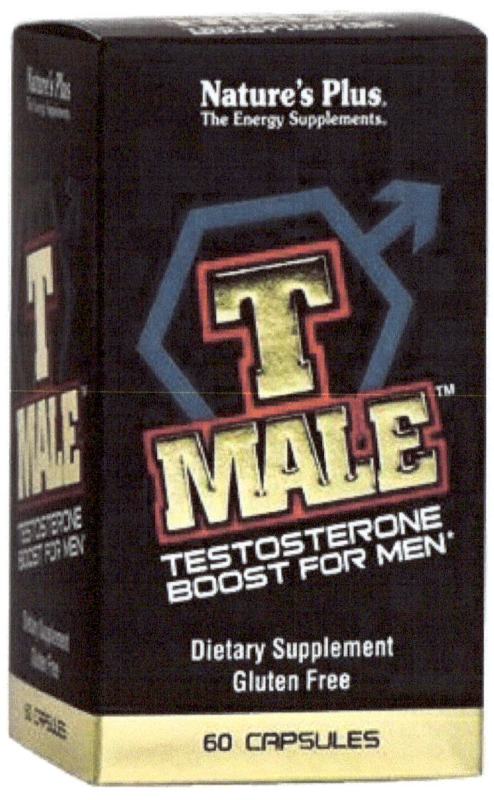

Swanson Testofen Fenugreek Extract offering 60 vcaps containing 60 servings at 300 mg per serving. This is a standalone supplement containing pure fenugreek extract standardized to 50% fenusides. This supplement really works and the price is very fair. Purchase online through Swanson Vitamins for $15.99

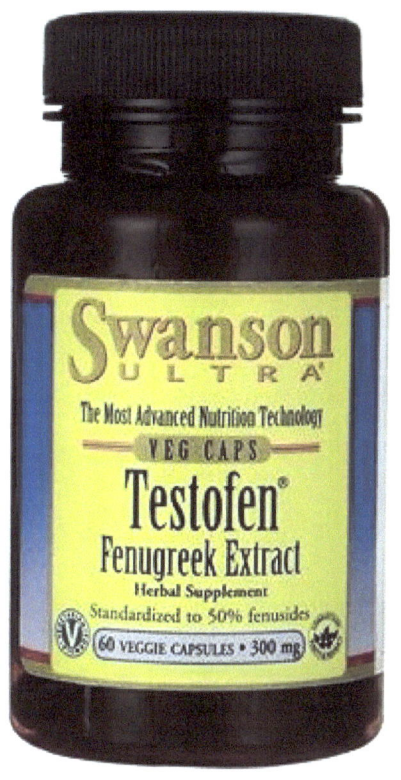

Universal N1-T Natural Testosterone Supplement offering 90 Capsules containing 45 servings. Contains a great combination of test boosting ingredients. Purchase online through Nutrition Express for $25.97

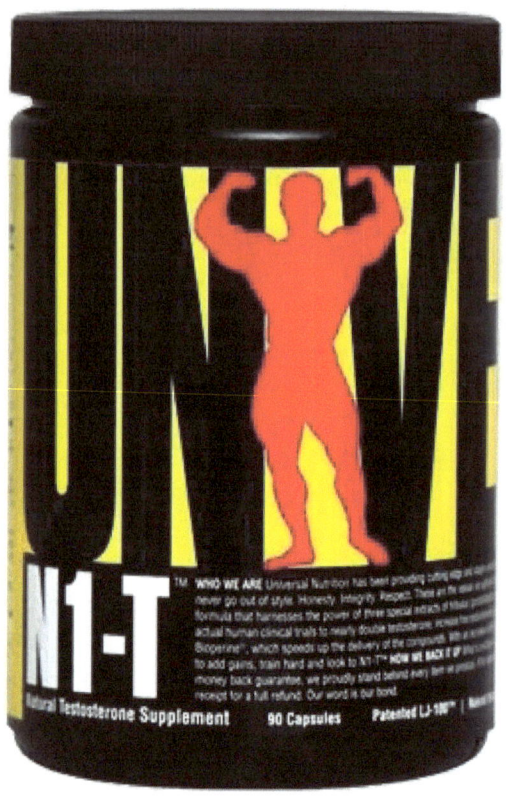

Irwin Naturals Testosterone UP offering 60 Softgels containing 20 servings. Contains a great combination of test boosting ingredients. Purchase online through Nutrition Express for $29.99

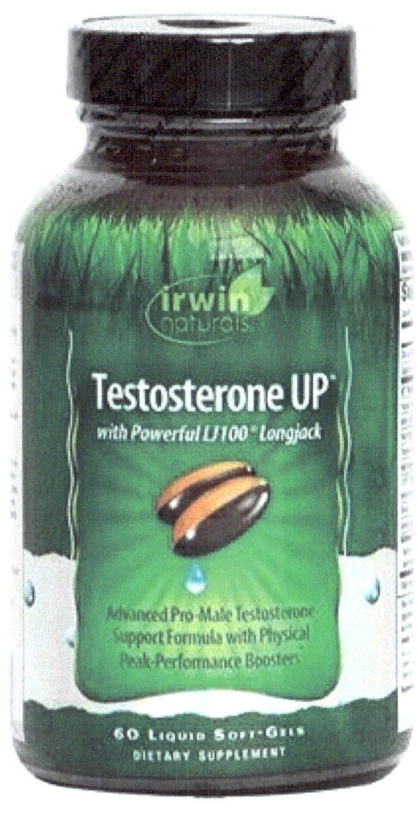

Nutraceutics Testron SX Maximum Male Support offering 60 caplets containing 30 servings. Purchase online through Nutrition Express for $19.00

T-BOMB 3Xtreme offering 168 tabs containing 56 servings. Purchase online through Prosource for $35.75

Androtest offering 60 tabs containing 60 servings. Purchase online through Prosource for $46.50

Androcept offering 120 caps containing 30 servings. This product contains L-Carnitine L-Tartrate (LCLT) at 2,000 mg per serving. Purchase online through Prosource for $22.95

AI Sports Nutrition D-Aspartic Acid offering 300 g containing 100 servings at 3 g per serving. This supplement contains pure D-Aspartic Acid. Purchase online through Nutrition Express for $21.99

People's Chemist Raw-T Testosterone Primer offering 60 caps containing Sarsaparilla, Fenugreek and Eurycoma Longifolia. This supplement could be the purest and best out of all of the above. I mentioned the People's Chemist Multivitamin/mineral supplement in my Series 1 book. He doesn't use any chemicals, additives or impurities of any kind and uses the purest and highest quality form of ingredients available. Purchase online through The People's Chemist online for $49.95

Pre and Post Workout Supplements

Pre and post workout supplements are basically powered drinks or capsules etc., containing ingredients that enhance your workout and recovery. They give you energy, endurance, strength, volumize cells, enhance blood flow and once again provide better muscle recovery.

NITRIC OXIDE BOOSTERS:

L-Arginine, Arginine-Alpha Ketoglutarate (AKG), L-Citrulline, Beet Root and Grape Seed Extract are some of the best and most common ingredients found in nitric oxide enhancing supplements. Nitric Oxide is produced within the blood vessels, which helps to relax and dilate vessels. This is beneficial for bodybuilders because it provides the volumizing of the muscles with blood and nutrients enhancing the "pump" and recovery. Some nitric oxide products contain Hawthorn Berry Extract and are really beneficial for healthy blood circulation and overall cardiovascular system.

My top picks for Nitric Oxide Boosters based on quality, safety and price:

Fitness Labs Nitric Oxide Boost offering180 tabs containing 60 servings. This supplement provides L-Arginine (HCl, Alpha Ketoglutarate), L-Citrulline and Alpha Lipoic Acid. Purchase online through Nutrition Express for $29.99

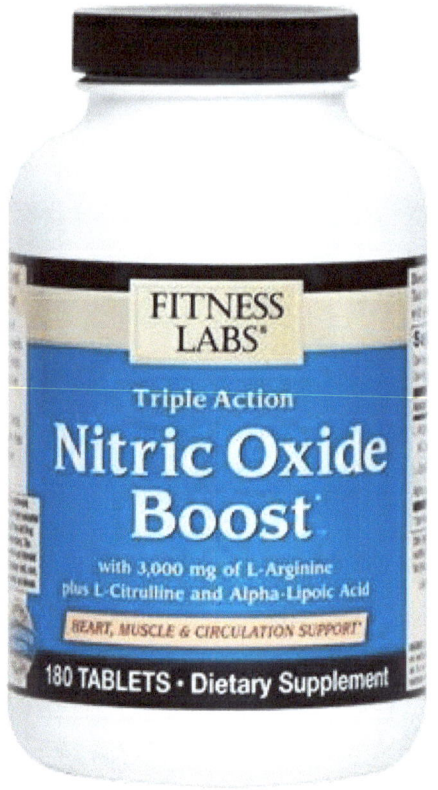

Irwin Naturals Nitric Oxide Pre-Sport with L-Citrulline offering 60 sgels containing 30 servings. This product has a really good combination of ingredients. Purchase online through Nutrition Express for $17.99

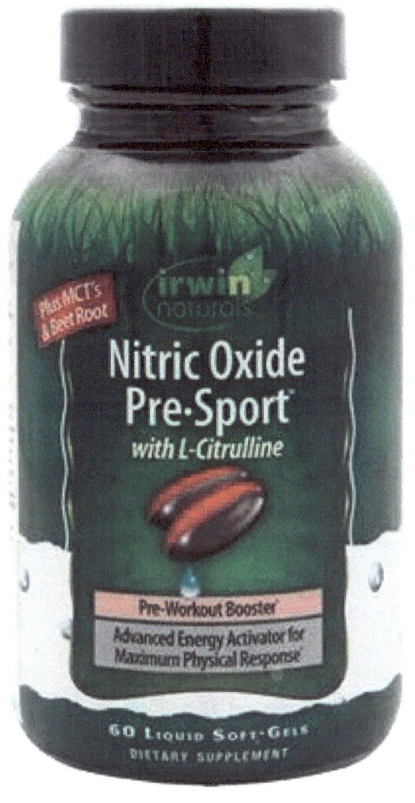

Arnold Schwarzenegger Series Iron Pump offering 180 g containing 30 servings. This dietary product contains a great combination of ingredients. Purchase online through Nutrition Express for $23.99

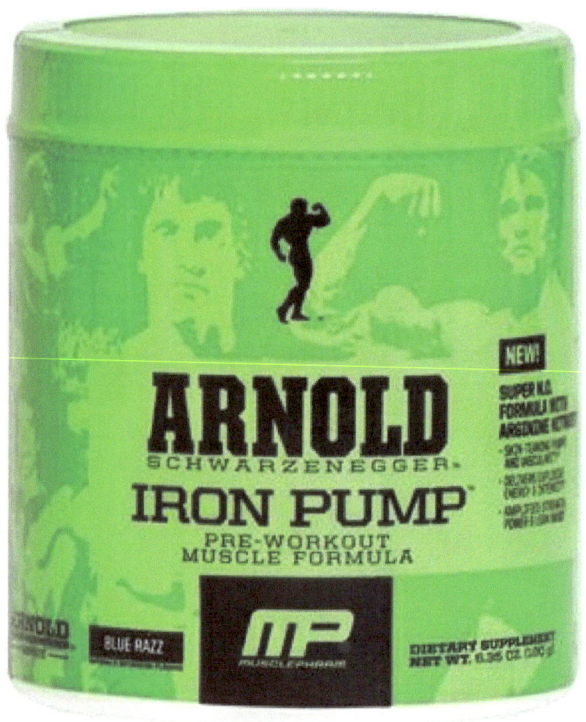

Prousource Super AKG Powder offering 180 g containing 60 servings. This dietary supplement contains pure Arginine Alpha-Ketoglutarate (A-AKG) at 3 g per serving. Purchase online through Prosource for $11.95.

Universal NOX3 offering 180 tabs containing 60 servings. Purchase online through Prosource for $27.95

Nutrex Research Niox offering 120 caps containing 40 servings. Purchase online through Nutrition Express for

$27.99

Cytosport Fast Twitch offering 2 lbs containing 40 servings. Purchase online through Prosource for $28.95

PRE & POST WORKOUT DRINKS:

There are so many pre and post workout supplements, powder and drinks on the market to buy, so it just depends on what you're looking for. I look for safer ingredients, less harmful chemicals as well as fair price and quality. When choosing a pre-workout supplement you want something to help give you strength, endurance as well as good muscle pump and recovery. When choosing a post-workout supplement you really want something that provides good quality protein, necessary healthy carbs and excellent recovery factors.

My top picks for Pre-Workout Drinks based on quality, safety and price:

Fitness Labs Pre-Workout Intensifier containing 420 g offering 30 servings. This dietary supplement contains a great combination of ingredients including L-Citrulline, Betaine, Beta-Alanine and AKG. Purchase online through Nutrition Express for $22.99

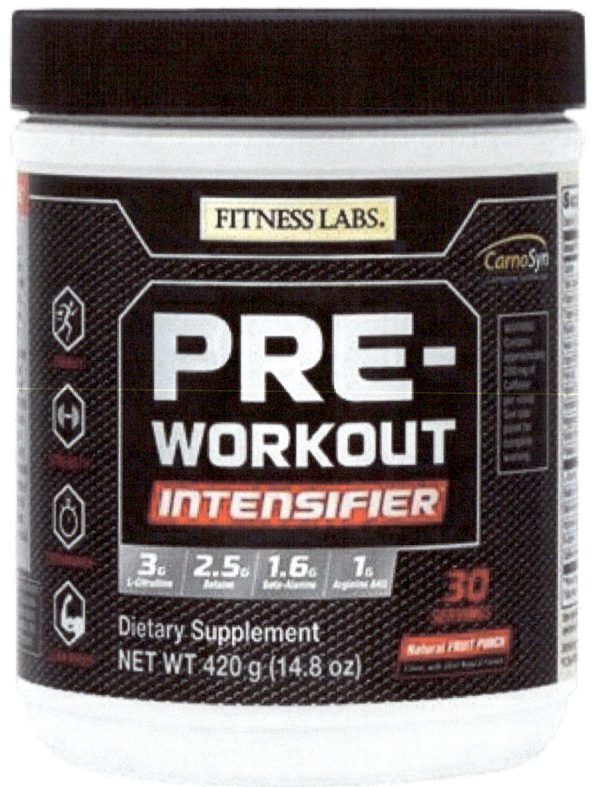

Beast Sports Nutrition containing 553 g providing 45 servings. Purchase online through Nutrition Express for $36.99

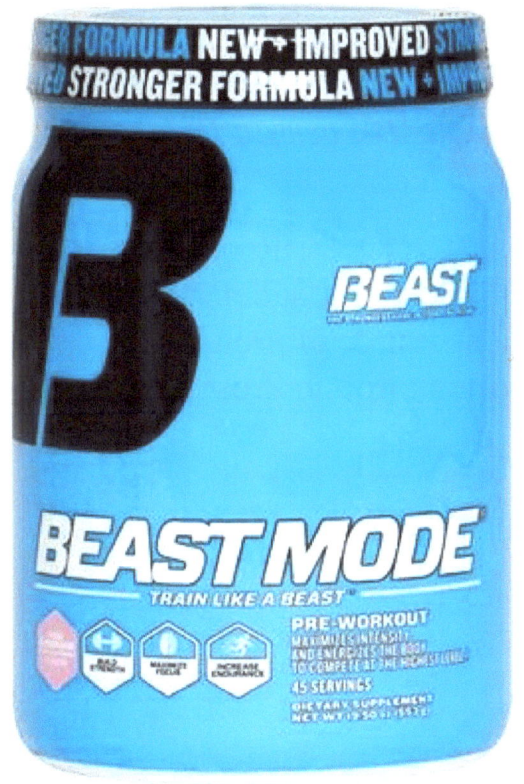

BioQuest AndroFury containing 336 g providing 28 servings. This supplement has a great combination of ingredients and was designed to also increase testosterone levels. You can purchase online through Prosource for $32.50

AndroFury does contain added chemicals like Red # 40, which may not be a big deal to many people. In my opinion, many companies should remove unnecessary

46

ingredients out of their products and strive to be more natural and safe.

My top picks for Post-Workout Drinks based on quality, safety and price:

Optimum Nutrition (ON) 2:1:1 Recovery containing 3.73 lbs providing 30 servings. This dietary supplement contains an excellent source of protein and necessary carbs. Purchase online through Prosource for $38.95

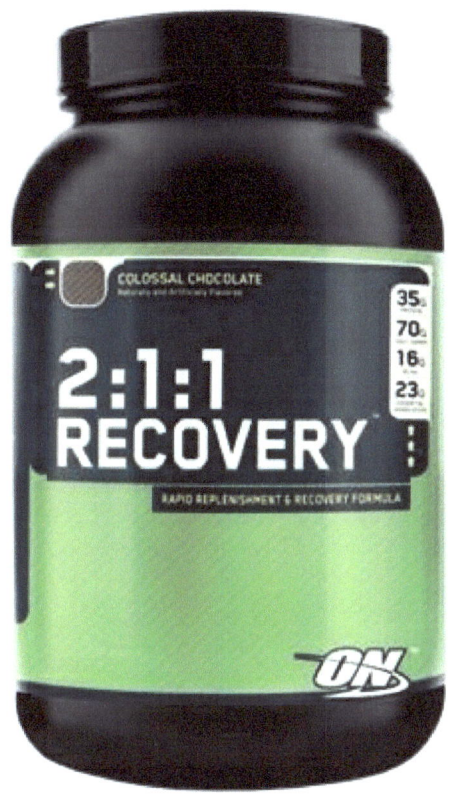

MHP Dark Matter containing 3.3 lbs providing 40 servings. This product contains a great combination of ingredients. Purchase online through Prosource for $30.85

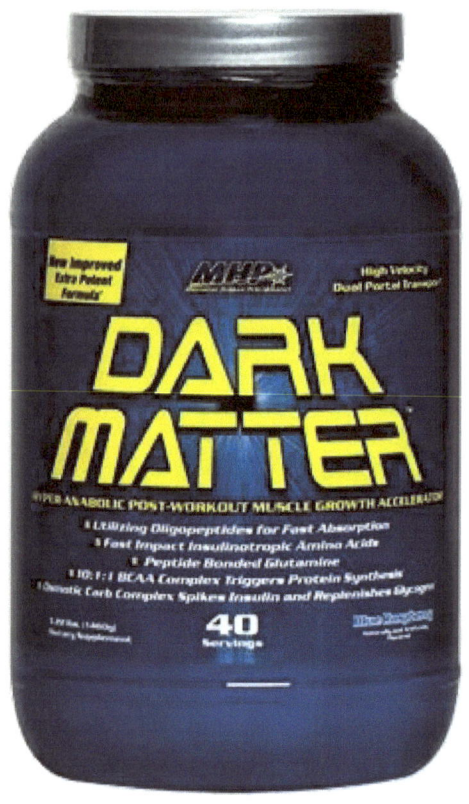

There are so many pre or post workout dietary supplements, containing creatine and Nos, that could be listed and shared here with ease. Popular brand names like BSN, Cellucor (C4), Bpi Sports, MusclePharm or MuscleTech have really great pre and post workout products that provide great results. It really just depends on what ingredients you prefer or don't mind within the supplements you use.

An easy and more economical pre and post workout idea could be just to mix some protein powder along with some creatine and glutamine into a drink of your preference.

Weight-Gain Powders

As an experienced hard-gainer, weight-gain powders are very beneficial, especially if you have a hard time getting the calories (protein, carbs & healthy fats) that you need from food. Weight-gain supplements can definitely help you pack on mass and muscle. At least today, compared to the 90's, there are actually some healthy good quality weight-gain powders on the market to choose from that actually provide good results and taste good.

My top picks for Weight-Gain Powders based on quality, safety and price:

Fitness Labs Gainer 500 containing 5 lbs providing 18 servings or 36 if you cut the servings in half. This dietary supplement contains some good safe natural ingredients and great taste for a weight-gainer. Purchase online through Nutrition Express for $39.99

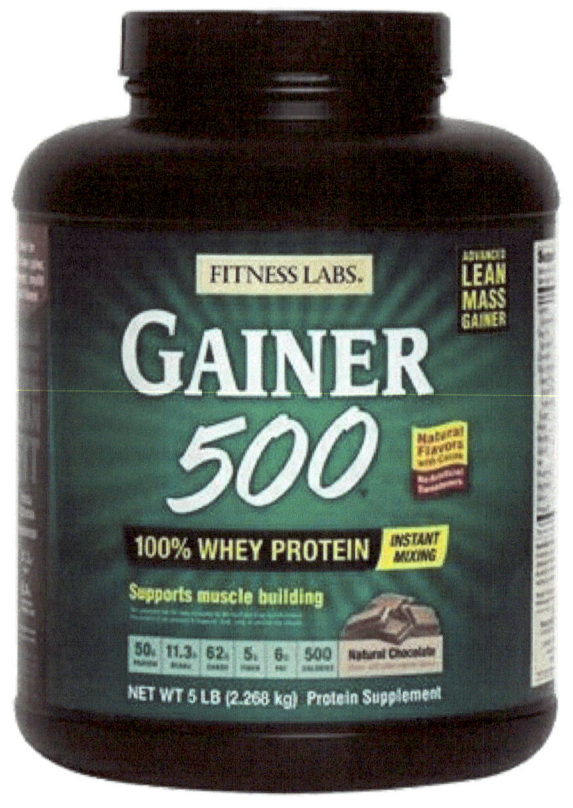

MHP Up Your Mass containing 5 lbs offering 17 servings or cut the dose in half and you'll get 34 servings. Purchase online through Prosource for $30.25. This product also comes in a smaller size containing 2 lbs for $13.50 and a much larger size containing 9.5 lbs for $60.95

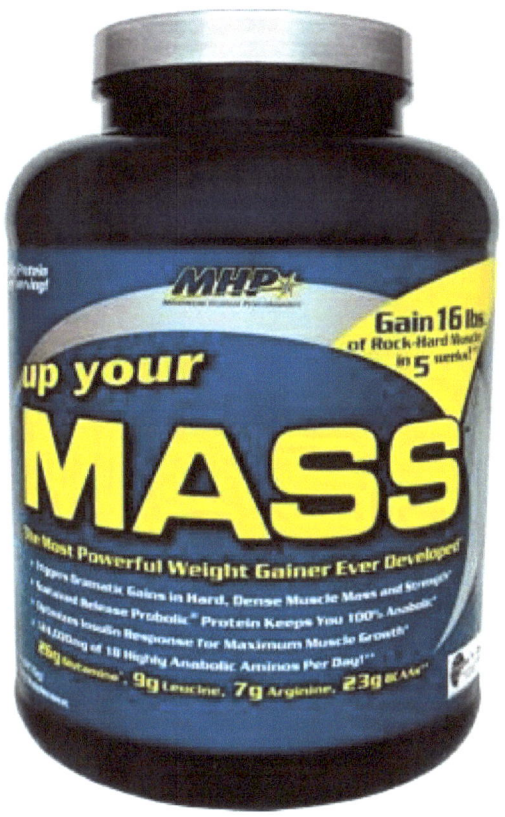

New Whey Nutrition Smart Gainer containing 10 lbs providing 28 servings or cut the dose in half and you'll get 56 servings. Purchase online through Prosource for $49.95

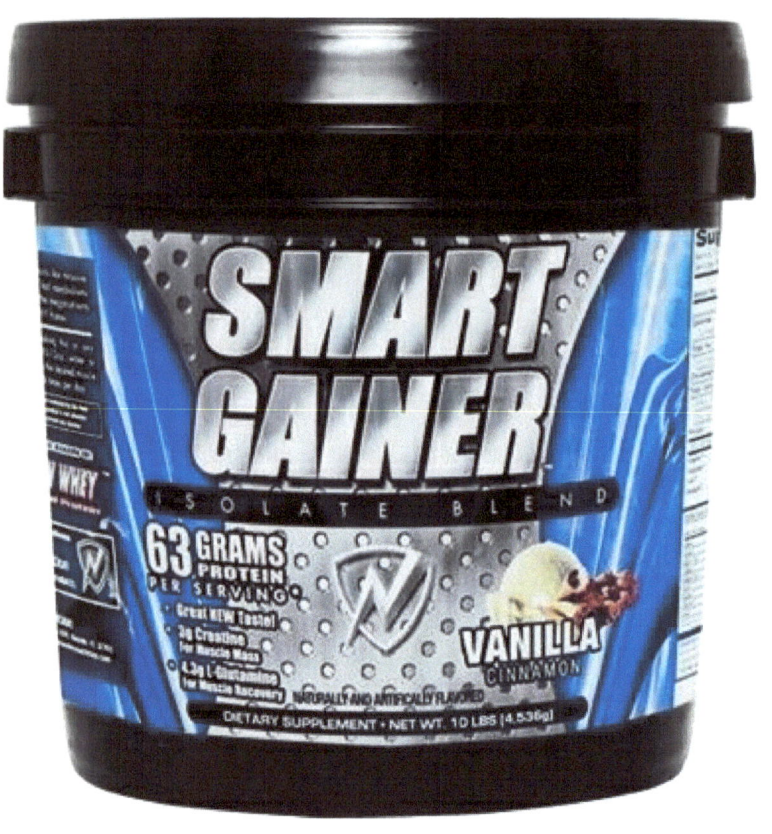

Arnold Schwarzenegger Series Iron Mass containing 5 lbs providing 24 servings. Purchase online through Nutrition Express for $45.99

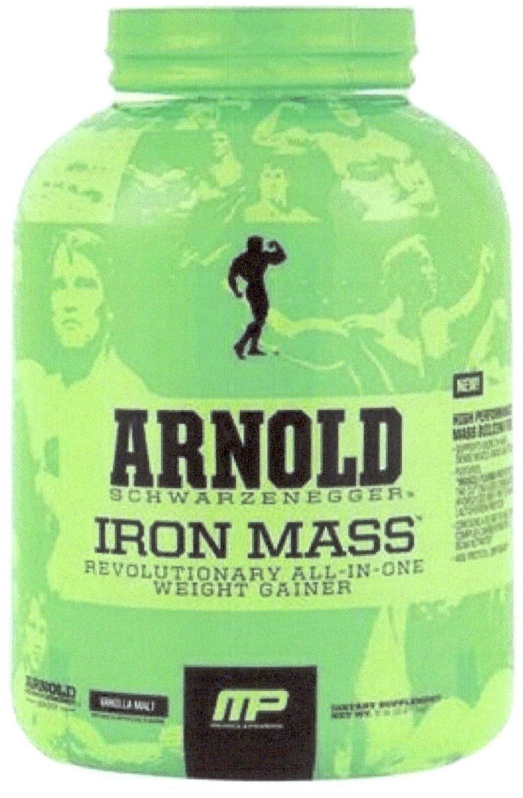

Cutler Nutrition 100% Pure Muscle Mass containing 6 lbs providing 15 servings or cut the dose in half and you'll get 30 servings. Purchase online through Prosource for $37.95

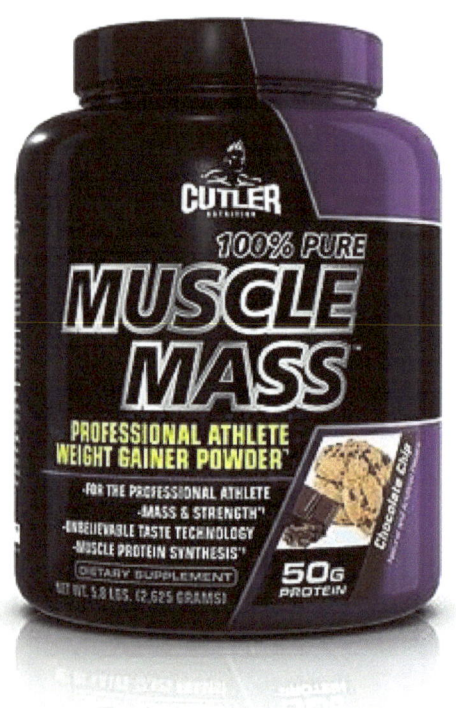

Bpi Sports Bulk Muscle containing 5.8 lbs providing 16 servings or cut the dose in half and you'll get 32 servings. Purchase online through Nutrition Express for $39.99

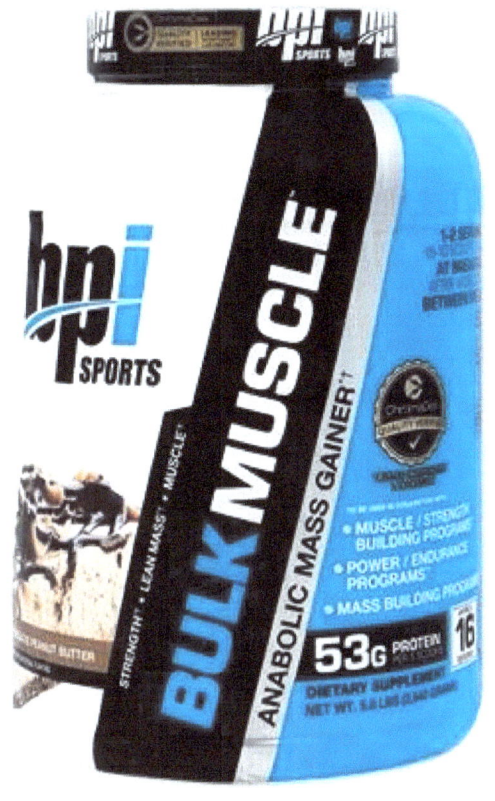

BSN True-Mass containing 5.82 lbs providing 16 servings or cut the dose in half and you'll get 32 servings. Purchase online through Nutrition Express for $45.49. This product also comes in a 10 lb bag for $49.99

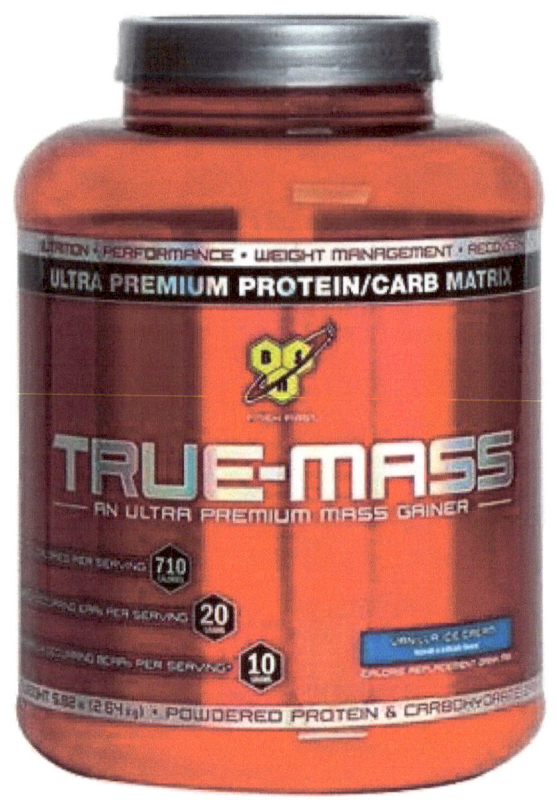

Part 3

Final supplement recommendations

Meal Replacement powders (MRP) and packets are dietary supplements that are beneficial and offer convenience. MRP's have been around for a long while but they basically provide a high quality meal in powder form, which would contain protein, carbs, healthy fats as well as vitamins and minerals.

MRP's, GH and More

My top picks for meal replacement powders based on quality, safety and price:

MHP Macrobolic MRP containing 20 packets providing an excellent combination of safe good quality ingredients. Purchase online through Prosource for $26.95

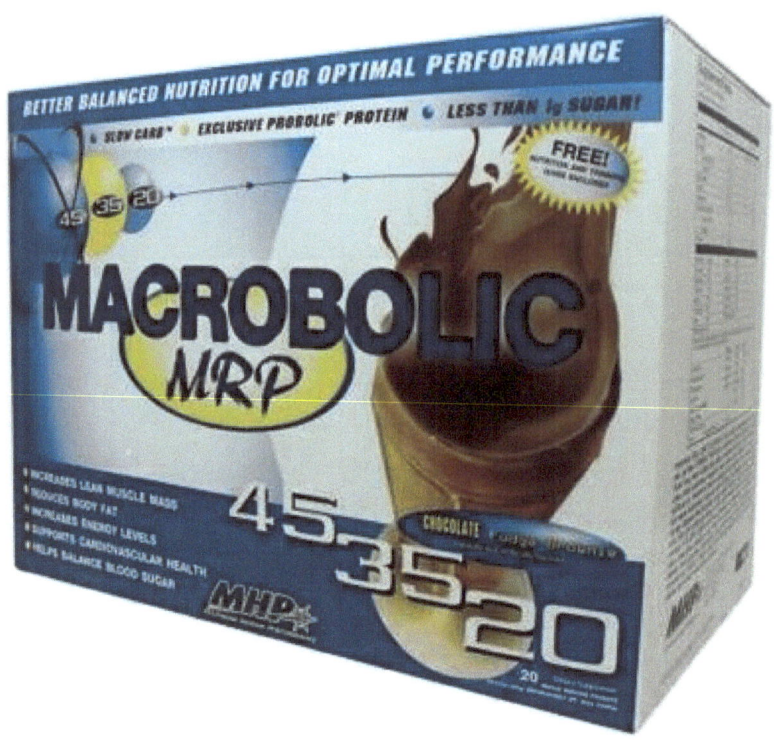

EAS Myoplex containing 20 packets providing an excellent combination of safe good quality ingredients. Purchase online through Nutrition Express for $37.99

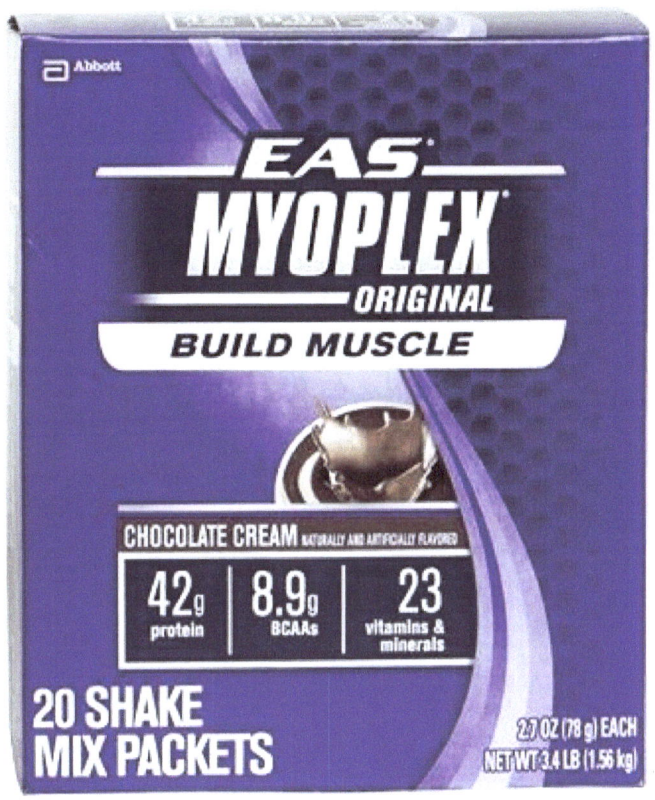

Labrada Lean Body containing 20 packets providing an excellent combination of safe good quality ingredients. Purchase online through Nutrition Express for $45.38

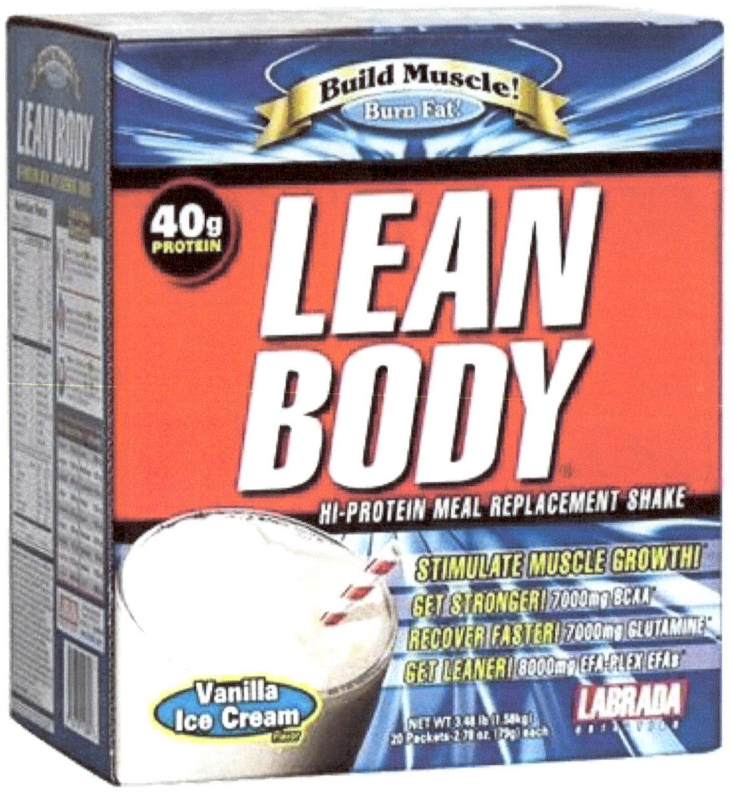

Labrada Lean Body for Her providing 20 packets providing an excellent combination of safe good quality ingredients. This MRP is specifically designed for women. Purchase online through Prosource for $35.95

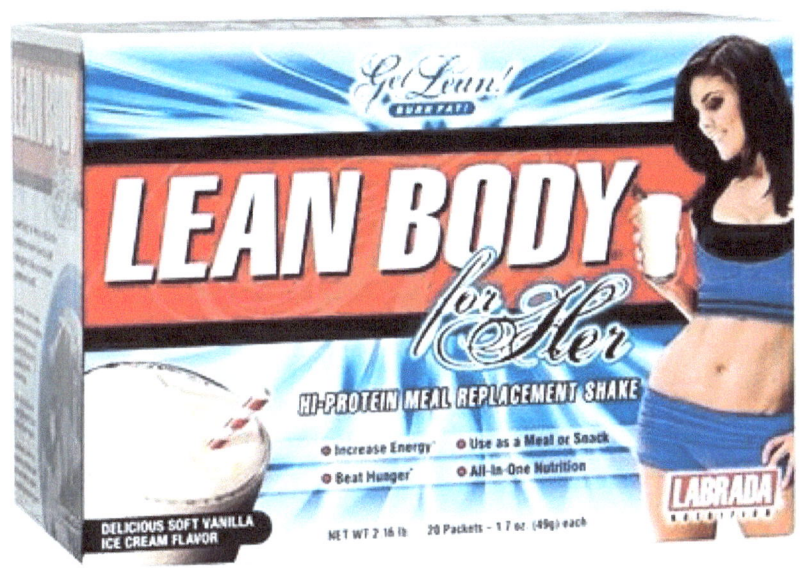

I also wanted to note that lifting weights is a great idea for women. There was always a misconception in the past that if a woman works out with weight she'll get big or bulky. This is completely inaccurate and many studies show otherwise. If a woman lifts weights she will actually gain lean muscle while losing body-fat. Not only will she lose fat but she'll keep it off longer, and as her muscles develop she will also have a much more sleek and sculpted physical appearance. Building muscle is key to both increasing lean muscle mass, decreasing body-fat percentage as well as speeding up your metabolism. Keep in mind that your daily food intake plays a great role in your success as well. Dietary supplements can indeed be a help and benefit in reaching your desired physical goals.

Here are some more beneficial supplement recommendations for helping people achieve their muscle building goals.

Natural growth hormone (GH): These type of dietary supplements enhance the body's natural production of Human Growth Factors and Insulin-like Growth Factor-1 (IGF-1)

MHP Secretagogue-One containing 30 packets providing an excellent and safe combination of ingredients for stimulating your natural growth hormone production. Purchase online through Nutrition Express for $39.99

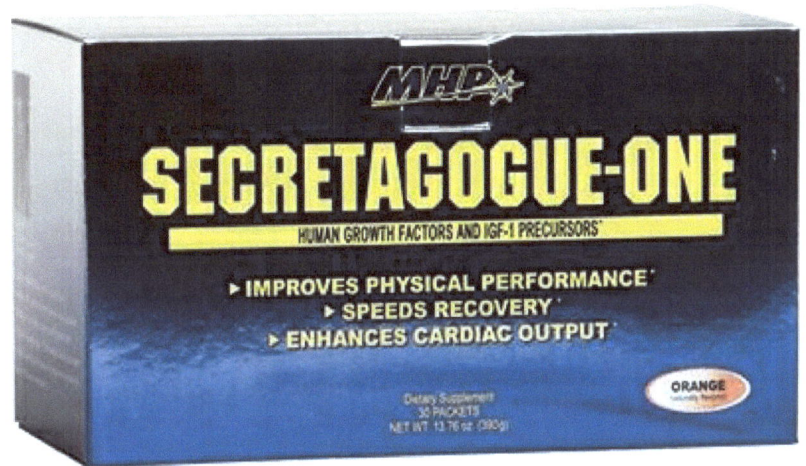

Arnold Schwarzenegger Series Iron Dream containing 168 g providing 30 servings offering an excellent combination of growth hormone and testosterone stimulating ingredients. Purchase online through Nutrition Express for $23.99

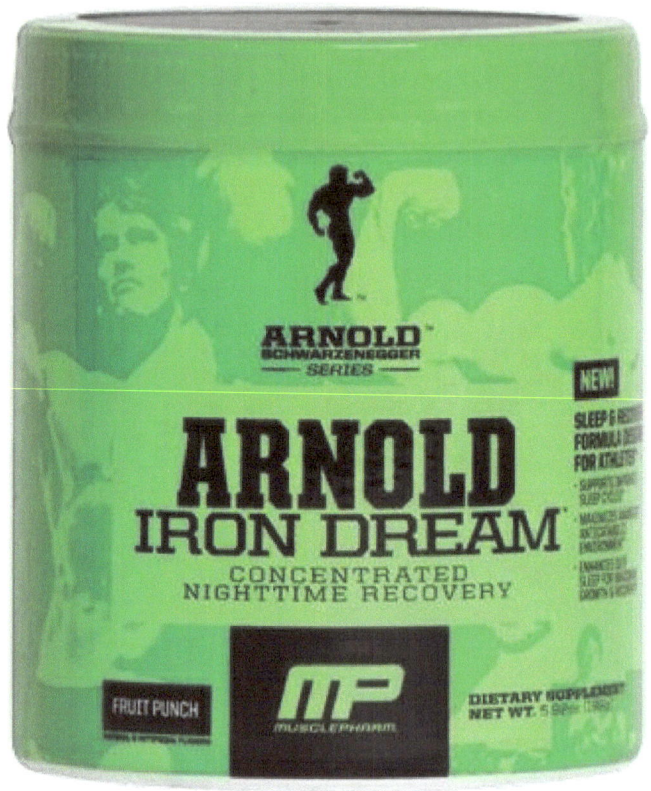

Prosource Dopatech HGH containing 250 caps providing 62 servings offering 2,000 mg Mucuna Pruriens extract per serving. Purchase online through Prosource for $22.95

Final Supplement picks:

Beta-Alanine is found in many top supplements that combine ingredients for optimal muscle building performance. You can buy this supplement ingredient by itself, which has been proven to be very beneficial for reducing fatigue, increasing strength, recovery and L-Carnosine levels in muscle.

Fitness Labs Beta-Alanine containing 120 caps providing 750 mg per capsule. Clinical study doses ranged from 3 to 6 g. Purchase online through Nutrition Express for $12.99

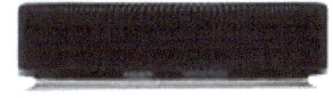

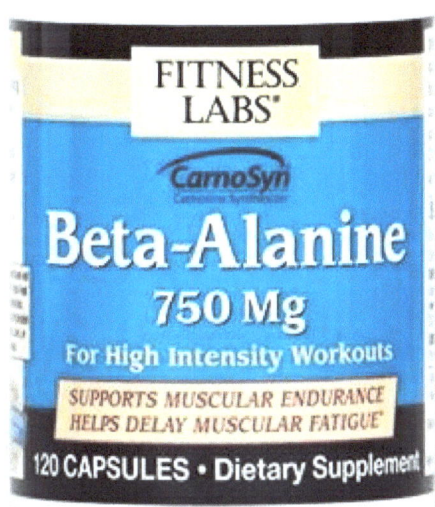

Fitness Labs Beta-Alanine powder containing 100 g

providing 48 servings. Purchase online through Nutrition Express for $6.99

Prosource Beta-Alanine powder containing 200 g providing 100 servings. Purchase online through Prosource for $12.50

Amino acids, building blocks of protein, are still a great choice as a dietary supplement for building muscle. Branched Chain Amino Acids (BCAA's) are key elements for muscle growth and recovery especially L-Leucine.

Fitness Labs BCAA fit 2000 containing 400 caps providing 100 servings. Purchase online through Nutrition Express for $23.99

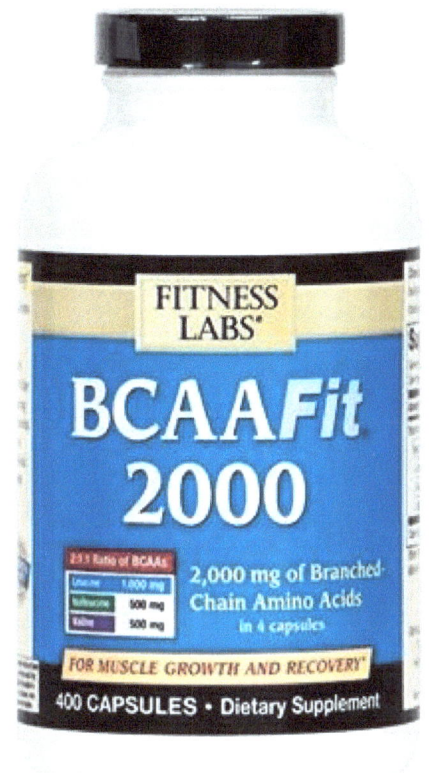

Optimum Nutrition (ON) Pro BCAA containing 390 g providing 20 servings. Purchase online through Nutrition Express for $23.99

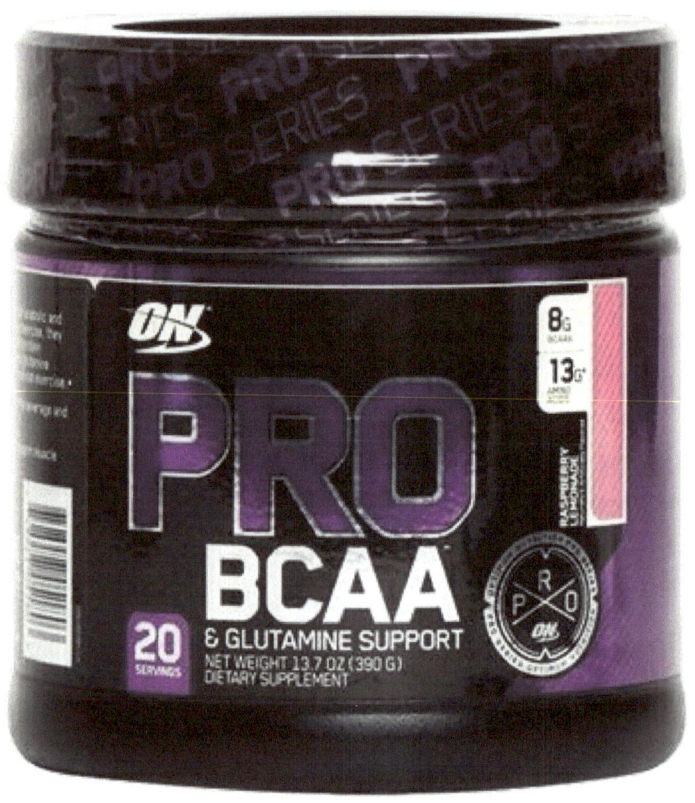

A few more supplements to include in your muscle building regimen could be Vitamin C, Vitamin E (natural form) and Turmeric (Curcumin). All of these will aid in recovery as well as help reduce soreness, inflammation and cortisol levels. In conclusion, building muscle takes time, discipline and consistency. Don't give up and I promise you that the results will come. Muscle building supplements will definitely help you achieve your goals.

END

www.ingramcontent.com/pod-product-compliance
Lightning Source LLC
Chambersburg PA
CBHW050811290526
45792CB00001B/66